C000116475

Move, Achieve, Inspire

Unlock Your Ultimate Potential.

William Lee

ISBN: 9798358894129

CONTENTS

SPECIAL THANKS TO

Special thanks to Beth Haughian and Selina Derby-Haughian for proof reading Move, Achieve, Inspire. Also to the legends who offered to cast their eye over the proof copies before this book became live to the public. To Marc Comiskey for the photoshoot that made the front and back cover, also to Dwaine from New Creation that designed the covers just as I wanted them to be. Moreover, to the endless number of people who wished me luck, shared my social media posts to promote it and to all the coffee shops around the town that allowed me to sit for hours while I wrote what was on my mind which is what you will read now. Finally, a massive thank you to YOU for purchasing this book. I hope it makes some sort of impact to your life, and please feel free to share it to anybody else who you think might enjoy reading it.

Please leave a review on Amazon, share your thoughts on social media and tag me. Once again thank you for everything.

William.

INTRODUCTION

Imagine a life not filled with anxiety. Life without fearing what people think of you and doing what you want because you want to do it; not to fit in or to please other people. To embrace your own authentic self and not be a chameleon by moulding your personality in order to fit in with the people around you. To me, this is what it means to be truly free. Free from judgement and ignorance from other people's opinions. Free to do what you want because YOU truly want to do it. Of course, I know it is far easier said than done, especially if you have lived years with the same thought patterns but with a bit of time, encouragement and repeatedly stepping out of your comfort zone,
 you WILL improve your way of thinking. It is easy to be trapped in our own thoughts and living in a constant state of anxiety, but the reality we create in our minds can change to a new reality - Freedom! Hopefully with the help of this book you will have a better understanding of why you have certain thoughts.

I've listened to a lot of self-help books especially during lockdown when the only thing we could do is go for one walk a day for one hour. I may have stretched the boat out and went for two in one day some days! This book is a combination of all the important parts I've picked up from world-renowned, best-selling books, podcasts and articles

I've consumed, and the knowledge I've gathered from working in the fitness industry for the last eight years. I've worked with some amazing coaches and have coached some extraordinary people over the years. From my experience there are a lot of occurring themes when it comes to people's health and happiness which I'll talk about throughout this book. This book takes away the fluff and goes straight to the point. I read self-development books, not because I suffer with my own mental health, or I am unhappy with where I am. Rather, I gather as much information as possible to help my clients and post informative content on my social media to help my followers if they are struggling with a certain area of their lives. This book may not directly be for you, but you may learn how to help your friend or family member after reading this book.

Nothing you read here is ground-breaking. Most of what you read you will already know. What makes this book powerful is that nothing you read here is personal, with nothing but your best interests at heart. I may not personally know you, but it takes somebody that is outside of your circle to give input from an alternative perspective to make you think differently. I'm not saying your current thinking is wrong, but shifting your perspective and ideas may be the key to achieving your biggest dreams.

Just like there is no magic, secret formula to dropping weight, there is no magic spell to living a happier life. You can read 100 different books about fat loss and the same basic message will be in them all - To move more and eat slightly less than what your body needs each day consistently. Same applies to living a healthy, happy life. No magic pill or spiritual wizard granting you special wishes involved. However, you can equip yourself with strong tools, beliefs and thought patterns to cope better when life throws all kinds of shit over you. This isn't a step-by-step manual that'll specifically tell you exactly what to do to be happy. Rather, it's aimed to educate you on ideas and proven techniques that may help you if they are applied correctly.

A bit about me

I'll not bore you with details of where I studied and how much "Passion" I have for fitness because literally everybody says that shit. Instead, I'll leave this part short and sweet. I've been in the fitness industry for around eight years. Fitness is my thing and I'm in love with it. That's it. Oh, I have a BA honours degree in sports studies. That always sounds cool even though I completely bluffed my way through my degree. Anyone I went to Uni with can vouch for that.

I run a personal training business called Move, Achieve, Inspire. My ethos is to MOVE more with exercise, taking part in active hobbies, walking, running etc to increase your activity levels throughout each day to not only gain physical health and strength, but also to improve your mental health. We must move our bodies if we can; to become the happiest and healthiest version of ourselves. It's so important to find what you love to do to have a healthy, sustainable relationship with exercise. Exploring different paths in order to find what is right for you is vital because a fitness journey must be enjoyable otherwise longevity is impossible. A fitness regime your friend is on will most likely not work for you because every human has different wants, needs and preferences. With consistency and hard work, you will begin to ACHIEVE results. Then, not only have you an interest in your own health and fitness, but you'll also INSPIRE your peers to do the same and hopefully follow a similar path to yours.

I honestly think I have the best job in the world. I spend the majority of my time with people who are in a positive mindset to change their lives. I learn from people from all sorts of fields with a vast degree of knowledge, hobbies and interests. I not only share my knowledge about health, fitness and mindset, but I love learning from my clients about their lives. I work flexible hours to suit me so I can take naps in between clients, have time to walk my dog and be financially stable to afford the occasional holiday or two.

PART 1

Identity.

Your identity isn't just your name, age, height and eye colour. It's your beliefs, your views and what you stand for. Your identity is what makes you who you are, which is what makes you different from every other human in the world. Change your identity and you will change your whole outlook on life. What's stopping you from achieving your most ambitious dreams may be how you identify yourself. Your limiting beliefs may be due to the fact you identify as an under achiever, or a weak writer, or maybe just not cut out for "It." (Whatever "It" may be.)

When you identify as a healthy individual, or a fit person, your whole identity evolves around that. It makes it far easier to maintain good health and fitness when you have this mindset rather than telling yourself you are "Trying to be healthy." Similarly, quitting smoking is much easier when your mindset changes to identifying as a non-smoker rather than somebody that used to smoke and is trying to quit. This is known as identity beliefs. It is far easier to change your behaviour rather than trying to change your identity. For those people that go to the gym at 6am before a long day at work and taking care of the kids must be "Mad, or crazy, or highly motivated." Or for those that still exercise while on holidays must be "Mental." Maybe not. This is part of their identity. This is who they are. This is such a massive part of their lives and no matter their schedule; health and fitness remain as their priority.

If you identify yourself as a lazy person, you'll create this narrative in your head that you just cannot do something because this is who you are. You'll never try to accomplish anything out of your comfort zone because you think you will always fail. This may be due to the fact you have tried in the past and failed. By slowly introducing new habits into your routine, you'll begin to realise that your identity will shift from a lazy person to a keen fitness freak, or even to a qualified veterinary nurse, despite the fact you thought you were way too old to go back into education to fulfil your dream to become a vet one day. I've heard countless times from people how they would love to be able to play a musical instrument, but they just aren't musically gifted. If you're passionate about something you do not need to be gifted, all it'll take to be competent at playing an instrument is consistently practicing. Learning different chords, shapes, strumming and plucking techniques are the only means of playing the guitar well. Some people may pick it up faster than others but if you take time to practice, you'll be able to master the skill. Anyone can learn how to play a musical instrument despite thinking it is impossible because of their identity beliefs. You do not need to be talented at something in order to be good at it. Practice will outweigh talent every time because skills are learnt and perfected which gradually improve over time. Do not let your identity beliefs hold you back from attempting something new. If you identify as a confident person that can achieve anything you set your mind to, it's scary the possibilities that will come your way.

When I finished University, I was completely lost. Throughout my whole life I was a student making my way through the education system, completing each year as it came and was always guided by teachers and mentors. After I graduated from Uni this all changed and I didn't know what to do with myself. I applied for literally any job to get myself off claiming benefits. I didn't have any ambition to do or be anything, only thinking about how much alcohol I'd be consuming on the weekends. Back then if I were asked to describe myself in three words my answers would have probably been - Lazy; I would have been too lazy to think of another two. Eight years later my whole identity has changed, and I am fortunate enough to say I am deeply passionate for what I do. I love my life which I certainly don't take for granted. Now I would describe myself as hard working, ambitious and with good morals. Looking back and cringing at your previous self is an important part of growing up. This means you've grown, changed into a more mature person and have adapted your actions for the better. For those who reflect on themselves ten years ago and see that nothing has changed are the ones who should be cringing the most.

Let's compare two different people. In this case let's say they both have lived identical lives, have the same build, body fat percentage, height and upbringing. They both have the same habitual eating patterns and are both overweight. One has an ingrained belief that he is overweight due to having big bones. He's lived the last 26 years of his life being overweight, so he thinks it'll pretty much be impossible for him to change. He has tried multiple diets in the past, but nothing has ever worked. On the other hand, guy number two understands he is overweight due to his habits and actions leading up to this point. He knows his body is a product of overeating and being too sedentary in his spare time. He too has tried multiple diets in the past, but he knows he didn't stick to it because he restricted himself too much which made him give up after a few weeks. He whole heartily believes he can change his physical body if he finds a fitness programme and nutrition plan he enjoys sticking to. If both these men started a fitness regime today which one would have a greater chance of success? Most likely the latter guy, right? The second guy does not have a negative identity belief which will restrict his progress in the future. He understands it'll take time and effort for his weight to gradually decrease compared to the first guy who would most likely will get fed up much more quickly.

Affirmations can be a powerful tool to change your identity beliefs you have used to labelled yourself for many years in the past. By making it a daily habit to say out loud that you are worthy, powerful, amazing, great at your job etc, it will distill this belief into your nervous system, so you not only say your affirmations, but you'll become them. Examples of affirmations you can say out loud each morning in front of the mirror are –

- I am successful.
- I am confident.
- I am getting better each day.
- I am worthy.
- I deserve to be happy.

These words will become part of your life because you'll begin to change your actions to mould into the person you want to become and not remain the same person as you've always been. Affirmations must be followed up with changing your actions because the act alone of repeating sentences over and over again will not change anything. Follow them up with actions that'll make you grow and develop into a better version of yourself. Over time with the help of daily affirmations it will change your identity beliefs into a more positive and confident person.

Your past does not dictate your future. For anyone that has had a hard upbringing, or has been in a long-term abusive relationship, or identified themselves as a failure does not mean this has to be the narrative for the rest of your life. The habits you create now and maintain will determine the direction you head. You should never look back unless it's to wave goodbye at all the shit you've been through in the past. How you identify yourself can and will change if you allow yourself to do so and not let the past define the person you are. Remember that the past is the past. Over time you'll have a different outlook on life to truly move on to be a happier, more content, free version of yourself which you deserve. You owe it to yourself.

For some people their whole identity evolves around their kids. Being a mother or father can take over your whole life, not leaving you any time or energy for yourself because your life is consumed solely on providing for your children. If it is somebody's belief that they are in this world to produce and provide for their children, then that is fair enough. But for those new parents out there - You are more than just a mother or father. You are still you, just with another beautiful, miraculous addition to your family. Don't forget who you are and your identity before you became a parent. Remember a happy, healthy mum and dad means a happy family with similar values and interests you distil in them.

Habits.

The position you are in now is a by-product of the habits you have formed over the last 6 months. Habits are the actions you do automatically without even thinking about and it typically takes just over two months for a habit to form. I'm not going to focus on the annoying habits you do every day that drive your partner or work colleagues mad. Like whistling along to songs on the radio, chewing with your mouth open, putting your empty sweet wrappers back in the tin, or leaving your dirty socks on the floor every night. Instead, I'll talk about the habits that are going to help you develop into a better person. If you are looking to truly change your life around, you must change your habits. Habits are the things you do every day that, at the time will seem small and insignificant, but continuously doing it for more than two to three months will then become part of your normal routine. Like instead of going for a nap after work, going for a 30-minute walk may not seem that drastic, but consistently repeating this action will become part of your normal evening routine.

At the time of writing this book, I have taken up an interest in running 5 kilometres once or twice a week. For me I prefer running on the treadmill because I like to see the speed and distance I've ran. Small, insignificant habits are like the speed you run on the treadmill. An increase of 0.1 miles per hour is so minimal, but over the course of five or ten kilometres it can be the difference of hitting your target and being off course. If the driver of a car increased his speed by 0.1mph you literally wouldn't feel a difference, but over the course of the journey that tiny increase will make the journey shorter by a few minutes depending on the distance. If running at 7mph on the treadmill to complete 10km it'll take you 53 minutes, 16 seconds. By increasing your speed to 7.1mph you'll complete your 10km in 52 minutes, 31 seconds. That's a difference of 45 seconds just by making a tiny adjustment in your speed, resulting in you completing your run faster. The reason why I'm explaining this is because if you want to make big changes in your life you don't need to make drastic alterations at once. You might not even feel like your habits are making any difference at the time, but consistently practicing these actions will pay off in the long run.

If you improve by only 2% each month that means if you consistently do it, over the course of a year you'll be at least 24% better. Changes don't need to be drastic, nor do you need to incorporate a huge amount at one time. People make this mistake at the start of their fitness journey and end up damaging their progress because they have sickened themselves or injured themselves by doing too much too soon. That is the reason why I only focus on one or two things each week with my clients. For example, when George hired me as his coach, he wanted to lose a substantial amount of weight which I was delighted to help him with. He began to explain his eating and drinking habits, and like anyone when they first start a fitness journey, he was keen to learn and make a change. He went on to tell me he has tried countless diets, exercise programmes, cleanses, group slimming classes and nothing seemed to work. Together we discovered in the past he always did too much, too soon and never stuck with anything for longer than two months. Together we incorporated small, achievable daily habits that were sustainable and enjoyable to fit his lifestyle. We worked on gradual resistance training and over time with consistently practicing his new habits, the weight began to drop off him and he was the happiest he had ever been. I coached him for almost two years and the habits he incorporated into his life then, he still does today.

Breaking a habit takes persistence, time and commitment. If a habit is ingrained in you for months or years, it'll mean trying to break it will result in an endless number of failed attempts to quit and take up a huge amount of energy. Anyone who has tried to give up smoking for good will appreciate just how difficult it is. Unfortunately, people wait until they are forced to stop smoking due to developing a severe lung disease, or quit drinking due to a mini heart attack, or stop overeating when they're told they need to go on high blood pressure medication. Why continue the route you are heading until you abruptly come to a massive crash at the end of that road? Life is short and precious. Way too short to not only reduce your life expectancy with your bad habits, but also the quality of life you live in the finite time that you have. If luck is on my side; I know when I get to my late 50's to 60's I will still be exercising, going to the gym and fit enough to continue to enjoy my life rather than being crippled by years of damage I willingly put upon myself.

People mistake commitment and discipline with being a miserable git. Like when you turn down that piece of cake in the office, your colleagues assume you're starving yourself. Or you must be mental to spend your free time in the gym after a long day's work. Or insane to go out for a run when it's raining outside. This is all part of living a healthier, happy lifestyle. Part of the journey you need to take to become a more confident, strong and content version of yourself. You'll be the one that is happy and comfortable in your own skin, not the one passing remarks about your kick ass habits.

Motivation.

Will power comes and goes like a wave. If you rely on motivation to do daily tasks, it's as mad as relying on winning the lottery to pay your bills every month. If you have started your fitness journey you might think you need a high level of motivation to continue this for a long period of time. It takes an average of 66 days for a new behaviour to become a habit. After something becomes a habit, it becomes automatic which means it becomes part of your identity. This no longer becomes a chore that you need to overcome which requires a strive of effort and attention. So, if your new routine is to join the gym and take part in group exercise classes three times a week after work, after this period of 66 days it'll be part of your weekly routine without any question. You'll not even think about packing your gym gear and water bottle the night before because it's an ingrained part of your normal routine. Or going for a walk every evening around your local park after dinner will become such an important part of your evening routine that you will feel incomplete if you don't do it.

So, what is motivation? To become motivated about starting a hobby, to do well in your job, to start a fitness journey, start meal prepping etc starts with inspiration. You may find inspiration from a wide range of sources like following the footsteps of your role model, seeing your friend doing a photoshoot which you aspire to do one day, reading a motivational post on social media, wanting to get in shape for a holiday or wedding etc. This gives you the initial spark which then leads to motivation. It is important to be surrounded by people who inspire you in order to develop. To physically surround yourself with inspirational people might mean dropping a friend or family member that is toxic to you. Whether they are bringing you down, or not supporting you, it's vital that you don't continue to spend the majority of your time with them. Energy is contagious and so is negativity. Negative people will not support you with your goals. Follow inspirational people on social media in order to gather motivation to fulfil your daily potential. It's important to be inspired by somebody who you look up to and would like to be in their position one day. However, you must also remember to be completely authentic and not be a copy of your role model otherwise you'll lose sight of who you are.

Motivation comes in two forms - intrinsically or extrinsically. Intrinsic motivation comes from wanting to start or continue to do something because it gives you satisfaction, enjoyment and excitement. You want to do it for yourself regardless of what others might think. You will happily do this on your own because you don't feel you need company, and you spend your free time doing your own research because you are genuinely interested in the topic. You'll want to reach a certain position in your job because it will be huge personal achievement as you've worked so hard since you began working there and you love the company. Extrinsic motivation comes from sources outside of your own thoughts and feelings such as a coach guiding you through your workout, not wanting to let your friend down so you agree to join the gym with them for a month, or a paycheque at the end of each month. For example, I was extrinsically motivated to do well in school to avoid a bollocking from my parents. Somebody might be extrinsically motivated to do well in their job because of the pay increase and the status they'll gain once they reach their promotion. Inspiration leads to motivation which in turn creates action which is the only way to gain results. Motivation is necessary to get started, what keeps you going is consistency, determination, habits and grit. It's important to have both intrinsic and extrinsic factors, but most importantly to enjoy the process and for long term results you need to be intrinsically motivated, otherwise you may struggle to keep going in the long term. If you are only extrinsically motivated to get in shape for a holiday, it'll be very hard to continue to exercise during holidays and when you return home. Therefore, you must find a love for the process or remain accountable for when you get home when your motivation levels plummet.

WILLIAM LEE

Let your own actions be your motivation. Physical movement has huge psychological benefits, but unless you make the first move it makes it much more difficult to do anything. If you struggle to get out of bed in the morning because the thought of doing all your tasks that day is overwhelming, then set yourself smaller bite sized tasks to complete. Tell yourself the only thing you must do today is your first task on your list which may simply be to brush your teeth. Tasks spiral together, and then you are well underway to completing your list that seemed so unachievable a few hours ago. You can go to bed at night and watch a highly motivating video or look up motivational quotes and be fired up to do X, Y and Z in the morning. However, once the morning comes that motivation most likely has gone. The best form of motivation is to get stuff done. For example, if you aren't motivated to go the gym, you can either wait until a wave of motivation comes to you, or take action by doing your workout, leaving you highly motivated for the next time you train. It's important to know that not everyone that exercises three to four times a week always feel motivated to do so, but if your habits, passion, dedication and love for exercise outweighs your current emotions of low motivation levels you will persevere. The feeling of achievement at the end of the day, knowing that you are proud of your decisions that you have made are the greatest rewards you can receive, and your actions will motivate you to keep the momentum through until the next day.

Consistency.

"There is only one way to eat an elephant, a bite at a time." (Desmond Tutu.)

In the case of this metaphor, an elephant can seem huge and overwhelming. If you tried to tackle the elephant by eating it all at once, you will fail. The only means of eating an elephant is with one bite at a time. Similarly, the only method of success to reaching your goals is to take small actionable steps and do them consistently so you are not set up for failure. If you constantly look at the top of the mountain from the bottom you will most likely get overwhelmed at the height and scale of it, making the task seem impossible to complete. Even before you begin you might think there is no point trying because the scale of the operation is too much for you. However, if you look straight ahead you may discover there is a path right in-front of you. The distance to the top has not changed, but now you can concentrate on tackling the path, only focusing on one step at a time. By consistently moving forward you will find you have travelled more than you ever anticipated you could at the beginning of this journey and the road isn't as difficult as you expected. Trying to climb the mountain as quickly as possible will set you up for failure; instead, focus on the steps in-front of you and with consistency you will reach the top and your goal.

Consistency is the key to success. Finding something that you love makes being consistent at a task so much easier. Taking one step forward every day is much better than taking no steps at all. Although finding what works for you takes time and adjustment. For example, somebody who loves to exercise first thing in the morning might be someone else's idea of hell and vice-versa. You aren't going to find what works for you unless you stick to it or try variations. This is the reason if any of my client's ask me which is the best fitness class they should do in order to lose body fat my response is always, "Find a class that you love and do it consistently." Trying a variety of classes will allow you to find the one that you love which will increase your chances of consistently sticking with it for longer periods of time.

If exercising in the evenings doesn't work for you, you will never know your optimal training time that works for you if you don't try it out. Too many people try one fitness class and throw the baby out with the bath water. Just because that one experience wasn't enjoyable does not mean fitness is just not for you. There are so many variables to life. Just because one aspect doesn't go your way does not mean you need to give up. Like having a bad driving instructor doesn't mean you can't drive, or a rude gym instructor does not mean the gym can't be your safe place.

Consistency beats talent. As Bruce Lee once said he does not fear the man who practiced 10,000 kicks once, he fears the man who practiced one kick 10,000 times. Going to the gym once gives you no physiological advantage. Eating one healthy meal does not reduce your body fat percentage. It takes time, practice and consistency to make the difference. Doing the same thing over and over again is so important to becoming better and to improve.

Going for a single walk in not impressive. An hour-long walk will not improve your physical health and you'll not burn a substantial number of calories. The same applies to going to the gym once. When you don't feel like going it is easy to think, "What is the point?" What is impressive is consistently keeping with your actions, progressively overloading your training programme to continuously see results and going out for walks even when you don't feel like going because the weather is shite. Getting 10,000 steps in one day is not overly difficult to do. However, doing that every day in one week is extremely impressive. 70,000 steps a week equates to roughly 55 kilometres! Doing that for a month will total roughly 220km which is almost half the whole length of Ireland! Now do you still think going for your walk today is pointless?

Novelty.

Novelty is the excitement of starting something new. After being in a romantic relationship for more than six months the novelty of starting a new relationship has gone, but you still grow as a couple. You still develop your relationship and continue to love one another, sharing life experiences with each other for hopefully many more years to come. It's important to not always chase the novelty to have a long-lasting relationship. This goes for not only romantic relationships but in your hobbies, goals and ambitions. If you always chase novelty, you will find it very difficult to stick at something for a long period of time. Novelty fades quite quickly so what keeps you consistent at your hobbies are specific time managed goals, habits and discipline.

As a personal trainer and a group fitness instructor I have demonstrated the same exercises hundreds of times over the course of almost ten years. I have explained how to squat and do press ups repeatedly to hundreds of different eager people willing to change their lifestyles. I have also performed squats and press ups in my own time over and over and over again. The novelty of exercise and coaching has gone. Yet I still absolutely love it. Why? Because it isn't the novelty that excites me, it's the passion to help people every day by witnessing positive change in people that drives me. I exercise because it is part of my identity. It is part of my weekly pattern due to years of practicing the same habits.

It'll be very difficult to stick with a new hobby or habit if you feel you need to rely on the feeling of newness to excite you in order to do it. Like aimlessly wanting to complete a 5k will be very easy to give up especially if you try to do it on your own. There are no consequences of giving up, nor are you answering to a coach or friend, so why continue when you start to struggle to complete your distance each week? Unless you have a strong reason as to why you want to complete the full course, giving up mid-way through is way too easy because there is simply no point to complete it. So how do you counteract the urge to quit when the newness fades away? Here are four points that can help.

1. Write down in detail your goal and when you would like to complete it. Set weekly goals to hit in order to ensure you complete your main goal on your set date.
2. Be accountable to a friend, coach or running club. By hiring a coach, it will

instantly increase your chances of succeeding due to being accountable to them.

3. If your goal is to finish a 5k; book yourself in a race 3-6 months down the line. This adds more pressure and will encourage you to continue your training in order to complete the race.

4. Buy healthy cookbook recipes, follow food accounts on social media or buy a meal plan so you are not eating the same thing every week to consistently eat well.

PART 2

Happiness vs Pleasure.

Happiness is a journey, not a destination. Thinking you'll only be happy when you buy a certain watch, car or get a certain promotion is a lie. Social media will lead us to believe that the wealthier you are, the happier you'll become. Wealth does not equate to being rich. Constantly chasing after material things for extrinsic reasons will make you miserable. Always feeling unsatisfied about where you are in life is like climbing an endless ladder, always climbing and looking up rather than stopping to appreciate what you have!

There is a misconception that money buys happiness, it doesn't; It buys pleasure. Sure, money will make your life more comfortable as you won't struggle to pay any of your bills. However, it is no coincidence that many rock stars and millionaires end up in rehab due to living the rockstar lifestyle. The money that they thought would make them the happiest person in the world can often lead to the opposite. Constantly topping up your pleasure metre does not correlate to happiness. Unless you begin to appreciate what you have now, you'll not even know what it is that makes you happy and you'll end up chasing an endless dream while being miserable on the way there.

Differences in happiness and pleasure.

Happiness is -
• Going to a job that you love.
• Coming home to a family or a dog that you love.
• Going for a walk with your dog.
• Going to the beach.
• Seeing results in your fitness regime.
• Seeing your business grow that you've worked so hard to build.
• Buying the first car that you've been saving up for, for the last 4 years.
• Leaving a toxic relationship and having your own independence.

Pleasure is -
• Getting pissed at the weekend.
• Having sex with someone off a dating app you just met.
• Upgrading your car from your old one that ran perfectly fine.
• Upgrading your smartphone to the latest model.
• Flying first class to holidays.
• Snorting coke.
• Going on a shopping spree.
• Overeating.

Find what makes you happy and do more of it. Simple acts like going for a walk with your dog might help you think clearer, brings on your brightest ideas, and fills your heart with happiness seeing your little buddy sniffing everything in sight. It may require a bit of effort, but the rewards are huge and ultimately make you a happier person. For me, weight training is when I feel at my happiest because I can really switch off, solely focus on myself and put all my attention into each exercise. This isn't to say that every time I go to the gym I feel highly motivated to do my workout, but knowing the feeling I'll experience after gets me through. A little bit of effort can go a long way, so by getting into the gym to complete my workout usually leaves me feeling absolutely amazing.

Remember you can only wear one watch at a time, wear one pair of shoes at a time and a huge television isn't going to make your TV shows any more interesting than a smaller one. The novelty of your new toy will very quickly run out and that pleasure you experience when you first buy it will run low, then you'll get bored and look for a newer version. Constantly chasing what you don't have is the opposite of happiness. Your thoughts are always consumed on what to get next to further increase your pleasure metre, not taking time to appreciate what you have.

To be honest I cringe quite a lot when I see someone upload an absurd amount of photos or videos of themselves during a night out. Especially those who depict how drunk they are and how they're having the time of their lives. This might be me being a miserable git, but I think the only reason these people feel the need to do this is to prove to their followers how much "fun" they are having. If these people are truly having as much fun as they say they are they'll not be on their phones. If they're as drunk as they say they are they'll definitely not be capable of editing a filter on them, writing a caption and uploading multiple photos during the night. Again, I might be wrong, but I think if you're sincerely enjoying your night out, you don't need to record yourself obnoxiously singing to Wonderwall on the dance floor. There is no need to prove to anyone how much fun you're having; just enjoy the moment with the company you are with.

The next time you scroll through your social media feed and feel jealous of how "happy" celebrities are in their private jets, in their huge mansion's surrounded by people, just remember money does not buy happiness. There is a difference between loneliness and being alone. Someone constantly surrounded by people can still feel loneliness if they don't connect with anyone around them. I would much rather be in my own company than to be around people I don't like. Just because you don't have a partner does not make you a lonely person. You are your own person; you are your own boss so don't let anyone tell you otherwise. I think it's a very old-fashioned view on life that you need a romantic partner in order to be happy. Yes, sharing life experiences with someone else is very special, but that's not to say someone that is single can't experience the same amount of happiness. Many people stay in their awful relationships not because they are happily in love with each other, but due to the fear of being alone. They may feel trapped because of the amount of time invested in their relationship, also they don't want to break up their family and a host of many other invalid reasons. Don't sacrifice your own happiness for factors like these and do not feel jealous of anybody else's relationships because you never have any idea what true feelings lurk behind closed doors.

Positive thinking vs. Action.

Positive thinking is like wishing and dreaming of winning the lottery. Or praying there are no weeds in your garden when your garden looks like a jungle. Taking action is getting weed killer and ripping the weed from their roots. Positive thinking is vital, as long as they are followed up with action.

Taking action is sorting out your overdue car insurance, getting all the necessary paperwork arranged and paying it off before your deadline. Only when you have your insurance done for another year you get to relax. No amount of positive vibes will get it done unless you take

ACTION.

If you have an ambitious dream but have no idea where to begin; just do something. Worrying about things that are 4 steps ahead of where you currently are will overwhelm your thoughts and make it seem impossible. Currently I have no idea how to release a book. I'm sat in my back garden just writing on my laptop chapter by chapter. I'm only focusing on making the content of each chapter interesting and informative, and once I get more writing done I will focus my attention on how to release this thing. If I were to worry about the success of this book even before I have written a word, nothing will get done because the anxiety of the future would determine my present actions.

Being optimistic about life is the key to being the happiest possible version of yourself. If you are optimistic, you'll ask yourself "What if my dream becomes a success?" Or "What if this turns out to be the best decision of my life?" Dreams only become realistic goals when you have a clear vision, write down each step and take the necessary action. It's vital you have the self-belief that you actually will be able to achieve these goals instead of spending your days wishing it would happen. Being optimistic means, you will at least give something a go like asking a girl out because you know there is a chance she will say yes or applying for a job because you know the company would be lucky to have you. Unless you're optimistic about the future, it will dictate your current actions so always back yourself in any situation because you never know what can happen when you try something new.

Change your environment to change your way of thinking. It's damn near impossible to change for the better if you are in a toxic environment. If you put a fish in a bowl of toxic waste and give it all the medication and exercise it needs, it won't thrive. The only way this poor fish will get better is if it changes to a new clean, fresh bowl where it can live a happy and healthy life. Too many people stay in their toxic relationships, friendships and jobs because they have been in them for so long. If you've to travel a hundred miles to your destination and twenty miles in you realise you are heading in the opposite direction, you obviously won't continue down the same road. You don't think, "There's no point changing now." Because you've already drove twenty miles down this road. If you are unhappy, it is never too late to change direction, no matter how long you've been on the same course.

Knowing something can be achieved is called possibility. Believing that YOU can do it too is capability. Looking up to role models is a powerful thing because this person has probably defined people's beliefs, has achieved far greater expectations to what others expected of them with hard work, graft and determination. If your role model is a professional sports person, remember they began as an amateur, but only their graft and self-belief is the reason why they are so successful. If you only believe they gained their success because of luck, this will change your beliefs that you'll never gain the same amount of success because you identify as an unlucky person. Only when you understand all the work this person has put in their early career will you appreciate it isn't about luck to be a success story. With true self belief in combination with action do you begin to believe you can also achieve the same results.

Confidence.

To me, confidence is having complete self-belief in yourself. Don't "Fake it 'til you make it." That advice is shit. Be 100% you, and if anybody doesn't like you then that is their problem!

(Self-belief VS imposter syndrome.) You may truly believe in your ability to perform well in your job, or start a new business, or become a famous social media content creator, or an incredible public speaker. You may have visions of yourself reaching your goals and have clear steps to reach it, but the thought of being judged might overwhelm you. I'll admit, I suffer with imposter syndrome. I believe

I'm a great coach and I honestly believe this book can help so many people. However as soon I publicly announced I am writing a book on social media I immediately began to have negative thoughts about people's judgemental views. What are people going to think about me writing this book? Am I qualified to write this? Even with lots of encouraging messages, imposter syndrome is still very much there. However, I realise people are going to judge you no matter what you do. If your self-belief outweighs the negative narratives you create in your head about what others think of you, imposter syndrome will not win. Having huge self-belief and a support network around you will guarantee you at least give it a go and if it doesn't work out the way you wanted it to, then at least you will still be proud of yourself. My self-belief definitely outweighs imposter syndrome. So the next time you're having doubts about a challenge or a goal you've been putting off for years, ask yourself honestly what is holding you back? Negative people will judge you whether you succeed or not. Having a clear plan will turn your dreams into a realistic goal which will further improve your self-belief so people's judgmental views will not matter. You'll be the one living your best life while the highlight of all those negative people's day is chatting shit because they're unhappy with their own lives.

You must prove to yourself that you can do

something in order to build your confidence. For example, if walking in a shopping centre on your own fills you with anxiety the only way your confidence will improve is by doing it. Only when you have proof that you can overcome your anxiety and the reality is far less scary than you thought; the next time you do it will be easier and building on that momentum until the task isn't so anxious. Just like muscles are built in the gym by repetitions of the same exercises over and over again, same goes for confidence. Continuously stepping out of your comfort zone or repeating the same actions repeatedly will improve your confidence over time. When preparing for a job interview, you'll get your reps in by writing down your answers to potential questions, standing in front of the mirror possibly with your suit on and speak out loud your responses. By the time the interview comes the hard work will be done, you've prepared as much as you could so the interview is the product of your hard work and the reps you've put in beforehand. If you admire somebody and wonder where their confidence comes from it most likely is a product of many, many reps over several years. Just like that guy in the gym who can effortlessly string out ten pull-ups in a row or deadlift more than his body weight is a result of countless reps under his belt to be able to perform those exercises with ease.

I think everybody has something they can excel in. Whether they pursue this or even find it is another question. Somebody can be extremely confident in their work but lack confidence outside of it. Additionally, somebody can be massively confident playing a video game but struggle in social situations. Everybody has a comfort zone that they can fully express themselves and be confident that they will do well in. You will never know what your "Thing," will ever be unless you try a load of different things. If you are lucky enough to know what your "Thing," is and enjoy doing it then I'd encourage you to really give it your all. See where it can take you. What's the worst that can happen? Find something you're passionate about and put your heart and soul into it because you never know where it can take you!

If you have the mindset of "I'll be happy when I lose 2 stone, or get a flatter stomach, or drop 2 dress sizes," I'm telling you that the happiness you think you will receive once you hit your goal is not as great as you think. Yes, you can cut out all carbs, not drink any alcohol and only eat chicken and broccoli, but at what cost? You'll hate the process and starve yourself for 12 weeks, hating every minute of your life. Your partner is going to hate you for being a grumpy fucker and your kids are going to annoy the shit out of you for even breathing. Instead, how about learning to love yourself the way you are. Yes, of course continue to develop yourself physically and mentally with training, exercising and eating healthily. Unless you begin to look in the mirror and admire yourself NOW, the process of losing weight to your goal will be hateful. Unless you learn to appreciate your body and be kind to yourself right now, once you do hit your target weight, you'll still look at yourself the exact same as before. You'll continue to shame yourself in front of the mirror because of a little bit of body fat around your waist instead of admiring your hard work and appreciate the positive, physical changes your body has gone through. If you've been hard on yourself your whole life, it's not going to suddenly change when you hit a certain weight on the scales. Chances are you were your target weight a few years ago and still hated yourself because you thought you were fat. Being confident means loving yourself regardless of your weight and being proud of who you are. What's really stopping you from buying that dress, or wearing shorts, or wearing a tank top to show off your arms and shoulders? I know your immediate response will be "Everyone will look at me and judge me." Honestly though, answer this; Have you ever looked at anyone wearing the same dress, or shorts and thought, "Who does she think she is wearing a tank top?" Most likely not. Then why do you think everyone will think that about you?

I think true confidence is owning your shit. The good and the bad. Always backing yourself to succeed in any situation. Using the doubt in your head to make you do better, not letting it cripple you and turning nerves into good energy. Confidence also means accepting feedback with real conviction. Knowing within yourself when you receive a compliment it is sincere, and you know it yourself without needing the confirmation from others to boost your ego. True confidence is not receiving any feedback but still believing in yourself that you are still a rockstar. Knowing that you are far from perfect and always striving to be better, but also realising you are worthy to all people around you.

Arrogance on the other hand is being told you need to improve and ignoring the advice, staying in an egotistical state of denial and thinking you're great, but in actual fact you're just an arrogant twat. Confident people still have doubts about themselves, knowing that they have areas to improve, and they reflect on their performances to make themselves improve next time. There is a fine line between the two but being humble and always being aware there are areas to get better at are the differences between confidence and arrogance.

The power of language.

The way you speak to yourself determines how you perceive each day. Turning your tasks into opportunities will dramatically change your outlook for your day. Instead of saying "I have to go to work tomorrow!" Or "I need to go to the gym!" Or "I need to clean the house tomorrow." Replace the words "Have" or "Need" to "I get to." By saying "I get to go to work tomorrow." Completely changes your perception of work. Your current job might not be where you want to be in a couple of years' time, but it means you are financially stable and allows you time to work on your craft with your side business to make that your full-time job. It also means it pays your bills and gives you the freedom to work on your hobbies in the evenings with your friends. By saying "I get to go to the gym tomorrow." Automatically shifts your mindset from dread to being grateful you are capable of using your body. You'll shift your thoughts from negativity to excitement and you'll look forward to the day ahead as a result.

The word "Diet," Has negative connotations associated with it. When people hear the word "Diet," They think of being miserable, being vastly restrictive, starving, plain and boring. Replace the word "Diet" to "Being on a nutrition plan." This immediately shifts your mindset to a positive outlook to your daily intake of food, so you have a better chance of sticking to it for a long period of time. People feel they need to cheat on a diet, most commonly in the weekends. You don't cheat on your partner every weekend (I hope), so why feel the need the cheat on your food? The reason you want to cheat your diet is if you're not enjoying the process or it's too restrictive. If you're on a plan that labels food as "Bad," then fuck that plan. In that case everything can be deemed as "Bad." Chicken, rice and broccoli can be deemed as bad if you consume too much which will result in you putting on body fat. If you plan your week and accord your calories correctly for the weekend out with your family, you can 100% have a bloody cheesecake for dessert and still lose weight! To have a healthy long-lasting relationship with nutrition, exercise, health and fitness you must enjoy the process. I talk about nutrition in more depth later in the book in part three.

When you're in a negative loop of thoughts all you can think about is the worst outcome. Consumed with making up negative scenarios in your head like being rejected from a potential partner if you ask them out, your small business failing or your partner not accepting your true feelings. When you are anxious about a particular event you should also ask yourself, "What if it DOES go right?" What if the interview goes well and you actually do get the job? Or you smash the presentation you need to give in work? Anxiety can turn into opportunity and hope. This interrupts your negative thought pattern, so they don't spiral out of control. The truth is anxiety and excitement have the exact same physiological effects on your body. When you are nervous about something, your heart rate rises, your senses heighten, and internal body temperature rises - The exact same as when you are excited. So, shifting your nerves into excitement will help you perform better and stay calm during the situation, making the experience much more enjoyable. Also, another question you must ask yourself is, "What would happen if the situation that you're worried about doesn't go to plan? If you end up not getting the job? Or the meeting didn't go as well as you hoped?" Life goes on. You should be proud of yourself for trying and you will always come out the other side better, as long as you treat it as a learning curve. You'll always learn more from your failures than your wins. The principles of exercise similarly apply. Repetition causes stress resulting in adaptation. Doing exercises causes stress to the body, but only if you repeat hundreds of reps of the same exercises, you'll become fitter and stronger.

Not doing anything should be an even scarier thought, so next time you are in a negative headspace use it as motivation to go for that scary task because the only option is to stay in the same position for the foreseeable future. Until you muster up the courage to put yourself out there on dating sites or ask that person out on a date nothing will change. The thought of inaction should be enough motivation to go for it because the consequences of doing nothing are far greater than giving it a go.

Speak to yourself like you would to your best friend. The way you speak to yourself can drastically change the way you view yourself and any given situation. Here are a few examples of how to change your language.

Example.
"Oh my God look at the size of my ass in this dress. I look like a fat pig! I'm definitely going to go on a cleanse after this weekend!"
Instead.
"Oh wow. Look at my ass in this dress! This dress highlights my hips which make them look incredible. I can't wait to go out and rock this new dress and enjoy my night with the girls!"

Example.
"Ugh, I cannot be arsed going into work tomorrow."
Instead.
"I get to go to work tomorrow. I'm so glad I have job right now, although it's not my dream job right now its forging the way for my side hustle to become my full-time job. Also, I'm working with wee Susie tomorrow, aww I'm so happy we met through this job, and I have built such a good connection with her.

Example.
"My wardrobe is full of clothes I don't fit into anymore. God, I have put on so much weight in the

last 4 years. I'll never be able to fit into these ever again. I wonder how I can go down 4 dress sizes in a month?

Instead.

"Okay it's time to have a clear out. I'm in a completely different place physically and mentally compared to before. Although these dresses don't fit me anymore, I am such a happier person than 4 years ago. This is what happens when you enjoy your food and don't obsess with your calories anymore. Looking at my old clothes is not doing my mental health any good, so I'll give these dresses away and treat myself to few new ones that fit me perfectly and I'll feel confident in."

Example.

"Maybe I shouldn't ask her out on a date. She'll probably say no."

Instead.

"Maybe I will ask her for a coffee date. I really like her, and I think she likes me too. If she rejects me that is fine, at least I know where I stand so I can move on. Either way, regardless of the outcome I'll be proud of the fact I asked her."

Judgement.

Positive people push and change themselves to become better. Negative people only want the world to accommodate them. Positive people genuinely love to see others develop and grow because these people are so sure within themselves, they don't push any negativity towards other people. These people support you on your road to success, and fully accept that temporary failure is part of the journey. They'll encourage you to pick yourself back up and turn that failure into a lesson. They'll give you the right advice to move forward. Whereas negative thinkers will only judge your actions when you slip and will judge even harder when you succeed. Being judgemental is a reflection on people's own low self-esteem. So next time you receive a negative comment remember this reflects on their behaviour as opposed to your own. You will come across judgemental people everywhere you go especially when you are on the path of self-improvement because too many negative people will expect you to stay on the same level as they are to make them feel better about themselves.

Always strive to be a positive influence on your friends, family and acquaintances. Nobody likes to be around energy draining people. Energy is contagious that spreads to those who need it the most. Having positive people around you is vital when you're trying to develop yourself into a better person so you should always distance yourself from negativity no matter who they are. Friends and family members can be hard to drop. Even though you know they're no good for you and the argument of "Well we've been friends for so long, I can't just drop them now. That would be wrong," is bullshit. Most likely that friend looks back from ten years ago and still behaves the exact same way. The person you were when you both became friends is not the same person as you are today, so why force a friendship that does not work anymore? A friend who doesn't support your decisions during your self-development journey is not your friend. The harsh reality is very few will give you their full attention and support, but for the ones who do; cherish them!

Elon Musk literally celebrated every time one of his rockets failed a mission to reach space. Each failed attempt is a lesson for the next attempt. He is surrounded by his team that genuinely believe in their projects to reach space which is the reason why after many failed attempts, he was able to continue to progress to make the next attempt a little bit better than the last, resulting in eventual success. If you are surrounded by supportive friends and family, they will encourage you to take risks, go out of your comfort zone and will support you throughout your journey. Anyone who does otherwise does not deserve your time and energy.

Be selfish.

Being selfish and looking after yourself is not a

negative thing. In order to be a positive impact on others, it's vital to put yourself first. Only when you take care of your own physical and emotional needs, you can then be a positive influence on your friends and family. When you don't take care of yourself, your mood and poor attitude will rub off on others. Positive attitude will impact your family's values on healthy eating, exercise and mindset.

When the mother of the family prioritizes her health and wellbeing; that has a positive effect on her kids because she knows the importance of exercise. Her choices for dinner will be a healthier option, giving her growing kids the nutrients they need to grow into adulthood. She will teach her children good healthy habits because she has more energy to go to the park and run after them. The shopping trolley will be filled with less junk food and more whole foods because she has developed an interest in cooking which has also sparked an interest with her kids. When a father prioritizes his own health and wellbeing, he will be a positive role model for his kids. He will maintain his health during his later stages of life to enjoy taking part in physical activities like cycling with his grandkids which he won't need to miss out on due to poor mobility or cardiovascular issues.

Learn to say no. Being a people pleaser is exhausting. Constantly having to go out of your way to do things because you don't want to let people down will drain you. If your friends and family cannot understand that you need time to yourself, or simply don't want to do something; they need to start considering your emotions and thoughts. Humans are not machines. We need time to reset, to rest and have calm in our lives.

Silver lining.

Devout religious people are generally the happiest people in the world because every day they put their trust in their God. Showing gratification releases dopamine hits in your brain which makes you happier. Christians show gratitude to God which makes them thankful for everything they have in their lives and even the misfortunes can be turned into a positive attitude because their faith makes them believe the outcome will eventually go their way and everything happens for a reason with a higher purpose. This isn't to say people who aren't devout Christians can't show gratitude every day and be just as happy. Show gratitude to yourself every day by reminding yourself how amazing you are which gives you chemical boosts in your brain making you a happier, more grateful person.

Journalling is a fantastic way to remind yourself of all the things you are grateful for, especially in the midst of hectic everyday life when you don't stop and realize what you have. By spending just five minutes of your day each morning or night will make you more appreciative of your life. It's easy to get into a negative loop, spiraling bad thoughts after one another and next thing you know you're lying in bed wishing it will swallow you up because you never want to get up. You can interrupt this thought pattern by writing down 3 things you are grateful for, 3 things you like about yourself and 3 things you've accomplished yesterday that you are proud of. Keep this journal and practice this every day until it becomes an integral part of your daily routine and over time you will have a whole journal filled with nothing but very personal reminders of why your life is beautiful, purposeful, and worth living every day.

How do you feel right now?

Being anxious about something is living in the future and not the present. Enjoying the present is next to impossible when your thoughts are overcome with tasks you need to do in the future like a meeting with your boss, a wedding you don't want to go to, a job interview or an exam. How many Sundays have you wasted overthinking about work the next day? How many meals out with your family have you not enjoyed because your head is in a completely different world thinking about work the next day? Or movies you haven't enjoyed because you can't concentrate with a million thoughts floating around your brain about a meeting in two weeks' time? What if I don't get the job? What if I make a clown of myself? What if I say something ridiculous? Or how many days out with your family have you not 100% enjoyed because of the dread of all the shit you need to do the next week?

Next time you're feeling this way ask yourself "How am I feeling right now?" I don't mean feeling anxious with your thoughts. I mean how are you physically feeling right now at the present time? Comfortably sitting on your favourite seat? Warm? Full from your delicious dinner you had with your partner? Sheltered from the pissing rain outside? That thing you're worried about isn't happening right now. So, focus on what IS happening right now. Be grateful for this very moment in time. Focus on your breathing, calm your nervous system down by slowing down your breathing rate which will in turn slow your heart rate to make you a calmer state.

The exact same rule applies during a long-distance run. (Long distance is subjective - 5k can be deemed really long to somebody including myself.) When you are struggling to get through each kilometre the thought of the finish line will seem impossible. Too far. Even unachievable. You'll say to yourself, "I'll never be able to do this for another 10 minutes!" But when you ask yourself "How am I feeling right now?" Not "How am I going to feel in 10 minutes time?" Your answer may be "I feel amazing!" Your heart rate is stable, your legs are moving smoothly, your breathing is steady so right now you are more than fine. When you are so worried about your future self, it will have a negative impact on your feelings right now which might result in you stopping prematurely, way before your physical body needs to stop. The more mental resilience you have the stronger your runs will be.

PART 3

Meditation.

Mediation is so powerful because it trains you to focus on one thing, and one thing only at one time. When you meditate your sole focus is on your breath, so if any thoughts float in your head you identify it, push it away then go back to only focusing on your breath. Why is this important? Not only does it give you clarity and calms your nervous system down by slowing your heart rate down; by learning to focus on one thing at a time helps with your concentration on everyday tasks. Just like when you're out with your friend for a coffee when they're telling you about their day, you can stay completely focused on them rather than being distracted by your surroundings or wondering what to have for dinner that night. Or during a meeting while there is loud construction work being done outside, you can maintain your focus to take in the information that is being shared in that room, rather than getting distracted by the noise outside.

I don't think meditation has to be in the traditional form that most people think about like sitting with your legs crossed, finger and thumb touching with the sound of waves in the background. To me, having a cold shower is a form of meditation that I practice a few times a week. When you are submerged in cold water all your survival instincts kick in; clearing all your thoughts other than focusing on your breathing to get you through it. Deliberate cold water exposure has huge physical and mental benefits that you can learn more about in Wim Hof's book - The Wim Hof method. I do it because it gives me a sense of accomplishment knowing I have completed something so uncomfortable and stuck it out. Although taking a cold shower may not directly improve your life, having the courage to endure such discomfort will translate to other parts of your life when you are feeling anxious. It'll give you more courage to tackle the big issues each day because you know you can withstand more hardship than you may have known. If a five-minute cold shower is the worst thing you will do in one day, everything else will seem easy in comparison.

Learning to focus on nothing but your breath takes skill that must be practiced. For anyone that struggles to sleep because their mind races with a million thoughts will greatly benefit from mediation. Learning to declutter your mind will help you have a better night's sleep, making your brain function much more efficiently and making you feel physically better. Just like starting any new habit, it takes time to learn how to do it right and find a method that works for you. Many people give up too quickly because they think their minds are too busy for meditation, but this is exactly the reason why you should continue to pursue the practice to help clear the thoughts in your head.

Murphy's law.

Murphy's law is also known as the negativity bias. Have you ever asked yourself, "Why does this always happen to me?" Or "The only luck I have is bad luck." Your brain is excellent at highlighting negative situations, making it seem that certain scenarios happen more often than it actually does. For example, thinking literally every time you go for a walk the heavens open, ruining your experience, or every time you order a takeaway, they never seem to get your order right, or no matter what; every time you are in a rush you get stuck behind a slow-moving vehicle resulting in you being late. You focus on all the times things go wrong, making you have a negativity bias with the belief that negative things always only happen to you. Chances are you have selective memory, exaggerating the times a certain scenario happened, making it seem to occur much more frequently than it has. An explanation on Murphy's law can be explained with a logical explanation such as probability, rather than just thinking you are doomed with bad luck. If you lose a sock, it is more probable you will lose another sock from a different complete pair because mathematically this has a greater chance. Or on the motorway you always seem to pick the slowest lane. In reality you only have a 25% chance of picking the quickest lane in a four-lane road. So next time you wonder why the world is always against you and nothing ever goes right for you, chances are because you are in a negativity bias, focusing on every negative thing in your life rather than focusing on when something didn't happen.

Let probability be on your side. One conversation can literally change your life. I know that might sound quite far-fetched or even farcical, but from my experience this can be true. Some of my closest friends I've made in university are a result of randomly starting a conversation with them on a night out. We often would have had discussions along the lines of, "Imagine how different our lives would be if we had never met." I've met many of my clients just from sparking a conversation with them either after instructing a group fitness class or on the gym floor. If someone gave you the probability that 1 in 20 Instagram post's results in a new client for your business, you'd obviously post as many as you can to get probability on your side to get more clients, right? What if someone gave you the probability of meeting the love of your life is 1 in 200 dates? Would you at least try a few? I'm not saying go on 200 dates because that'll be exhausting and expensive, but when it's pitched to you like this, the anxiety of asking someone out wouldn't be so daunting. The fear of rejection will also decrease because you know the chances of it working out were quite slim in the first place. When it comes to business you can't let the fear of rejection get in your way. Offering your services to as many people as possible will result in a lot of rejections, but out of them hundreds of rejections will be a keen client willing to hire you. Getting probability on your side is like buying yourself lottery tickets. It may work out, it may not; but at least you've increased your chances of winning even if the chances are slim.

Toxic motivation.

How many social media posts have you seen personal trainers caption their photos with "No excuses!" Or "Never skip a Monday!" Firstly, who is anybody to tell you if your "Excuse," for not attending the gym is valid or not? There are plenty of reasons doing your workout might have not been possible that day. All these posts do is spread guilt to those who read them - not motivation to persuade the reader to go to the gym. The stigma of never missing a Monday, I think is absolute shite. The start of the week is not the same for everyone! It's damaging to have this mindset because if Monday comes and goes without getting your workout in, then what? Do you wait until the next week? This is where quotes like "Diet starts on Monday," (When it is only Tuesday come from!)

Instead of thinking you need to have a good start to the week in order to build on that momentum to carry you on the rest of the week, think about ending your week on a high. Switch your mindset to think "Okay, it's Friday and I still haven't been to the gym yet or tracked my calories. At least I will have three days to get a bit done before the week is up. By starting today, it will be far less of a challenge come Monday to make up for the whole week off track."

Toxic motivation comes in all forms, not just the gym environment. It seems the harder someone works, the less sleep they get and more energy drinks they consume; the more attention on social media they get. Sleeping for four hours, working for eighteen hours, and working out for two just isn't realistic for everybody. It's entertaining as hell to watch though. What becomes toxic is when young people see this and think the only way they will become successful is living this lifestyle. What can happen is young people don't think they have what it takes to become like these people, so why even try? It's so important to not only surround yourself with positive people, but flood your social media feed with people that will lift your mood rather than bring you down.

Success.

Throughout my childhood when I was in school my success as a student was determined solely on my grades. Kids are taught to believe that if they don't achieve the grades their teachers set them up for, they will struggle to get into university, thus making them a failure because they will not have a "Successful" job. What this means is you won't be an employee for a top firm, working miserable hours for a boss or company that does not give a shit about you whilst paying back a student loan that'll make you cry at the thought of. Just because you wear a suit, tie and fancy trousers every day does not make you successful! Remember employees are employed to do the most amount of work for the least amount of money possible.

What does it mean to be successful? A well-paid job? Wearing designer shoes? Earning a certain salary a month to buy a car and house that's too big for your lonely ass? I would much rather earn a significantly less amount in exchange for a happy working life in addition to a fulfilled life full of adventures, laughter, reduced stress and sleeping at night without worrying about the next day. It makes me so sad to think the majority of people's lives are based around their hatred of the weekdays, and the only real happiness they experience is at the weekends when they don't need to worry about work. Even at that, Sundays are filled with dread because they know the next day, they need to return to that hell hole that is their office to sit beside fucking Karen who will moan about her awful relationship and Jimmy who complains about being out of breath going to the vending machine for his 2nd snickers bar before 12pm.

To me, success is not how many grades you have, or the car you drive, or how many suits you own. To be honest, success is completely subjective. As a fitness coach for the last eight years, I have helped a lot of people with a vast degree of goals and success. To some, simply even stepping into the gym to chat with me has been a massive win. Completing a 5k race without stopping is success. Performing 5 press ups in a row for the first time is a huge victory. If success means to you not having a panic attack going into the hairdressers by yourself, fucking celebrate it! Don't let anybody determine what success means to you. If you are proud of your wins then that's all that matters.

The fitness industry.

For anybody thinking of starting a career in the fitness industry, I would strongly recommend you go for it. If one of your limiting beliefs is that you'll not succeed because the industry is saturated, you're absolutely right. If you do what every other

PT does, you'll get lost in the crowd. If you don't stand out with your brand and give people a reason to hire you as their coach, you will struggle to get your feet off the ground. Why try to be like everyone else when everybody else is taken? Be unapologetically you. Be as authentic as you can because trying to be somebody you are not is exhausting. This not only applies to the fitness industry. For anybody considering working for themselves, take the right steps to get you to where you would love to be!

For anybody in the position that is looking to hire a fitness coach to help them achieve their goals here are a few pointers to look out for.

- Just because somebody has an amazing body it does not make them a good coach! Somebody who has gone through a twelve-week transformation and has achieved amazing results from it does not mean they know how to help YOU achieve the same results. Body builders that have an amazing physique know exactly how to get their own body the optimal best with the help of a coach. Remember body building is a sport that requires an extraordinary amount of time, dedication, sacrifice and good genetics. This doesn't qualify them as a good coach and know the best way to help the general population.

- Meet up with a potential coach before you decide to hire them. I always make it a priority to meet my clients before we work together because I understand the importance of building a connection with my clients. Any coach that can't dedicate ten minutes to meet for a chat before you hire them does not value your time. All they care about is your money.

- Hire a coach that you know has genuinely helped people. Somebody that has good reviews, posts transformations or you know they have a good reputation.

Hiring a coach has endless benefits to help you push you to where you want to be. The accountability of having a coach pushes you far more than doing it yourself. However not everybody is in the position to hire a coach and don't have a partner to accompany them to the gym. So, the only other option is to do it alone.

Walking in a gym for the first time alone is daunting and all you can think about is, "Why is everyone staring at me?!" Anxiety may creep in and all you want to do is leave. Instead of looking around you at all these seemingly amazing, fit and strong professional lifters around you, try to look past their exterior being. The person beside you with layers of muscles on top of more layers of muscle may be feeling the exact same way. That person may be a stressed-out father who is working long, boring shifts and this is his only time for himself. The lady you see with the "Perfect figure," has most likely been working on her craft for several years with plenty of ups and downs along the way. Most likely these people are only concentrating on their own workout and nothing else.

Everyone is on their own journey; the gym is not a place to judge but a place to help build people physically and mentally. Look past the size of someone's bicep and admire their determination, personality and passion.

Here are a few tips to help you overcome your fear of going into the gym yourself.

1. Have a very clear idea what you are going to do. Get somebody to write you out a program or write one yourself. Keep it short and sweet. Study it before you leave the house and know exactly what you are going to do.

2. Confidence is built on acts of courage. Taking the first step and stepping foot into the gym on your own will build on your confidence for the next time you go in. Prove to yourself it isn't so bad!

3. Stick on your headphones and zone out. Visualise yourself in your own little bubble. It does not matter if there are only four people or forty people around you, focus on your bubble. Nobody is looking at you or judging you. If you are on the treadmill that is your bubble. If you are on the lat pulldown machine you are in that bubble.

4. Be fucking proud of yourself when you get in there! It's definitely no easy feat so celebrate to yourself!

Nutrition 101.

If you are looking to lose body fat the only way you will achieve this is with a calorie deficit. This means you must eat, and drink less than you burn. You can do this by reducing the number of calories you consume, or increase your energy expenditure each day, or better yet - both! No training programme will outweigh a bad diet which means you can work your ass off in the gym but still not lose any weight because you are still consuming more calories than you need. Going to the gym to burn calories really isn't the answer. Have you ever looked at the calories burned when on a treadmill or cross trainer after 30 minutes of hard work? The number of calories you burn is depressingly low for the amount of work you have put in. If you try to burn off all the calories you eat, you will literally work yourself to the ground. The majority of the calories you burn in a daily basis do not come from the gym, rather it comes from the tasks you do the rest of the day called non exercise activity thermogenesis - NEAT. Examples of NEAT are brushing your teeth, walking to the shop, walking your dog, doing laundry, walking up the steps, walking around the shops. The higher your activity levels, the more calories you will burn throughout the day, thus putting you in more of a calorie deficit to lose excess body fat. It is highly possible to lose weight by solely reducing the calories you eat, however by adding resistance training you are not only burning calories, but you are also changing the structure of your body called body recomposition. Weight training builds muscle which, with consistency and progressive overload (Progressively making your programme harder each week), You are changing the way you look and feel. You will build a solid, strong and healthy body that you can be proud of.

Calories are broken down into categories called macronutrients and micronutrients. Micronutrients are included in vitamins and minerals which are vital for growth, immune function and brain development. There are three macronutrients: protein, fats and carbohydrates. All of these have a different role to play to have a healthy functioning body especially for anybody putting their body under controlled stress like weight training a few times a week. Protein helps build and repair muscles providing 4 calories per gram. Carbohydrates fuel our bodies with energy providing 4 calories per gram. Fats help us stay warm, provide energy and helps absorb vitamins, providing 9 calories per gram. Weight loss and weight gain is solely dictated by food and drink QUANTITY; however, food and drink QUALITY dictate your health. If you cut out all carbohydrates in your diet but are still eating more calories than you burn, then you will put on body fat. Same goes for any macronutrients. Cutting out fats from your diet will not necessarily mean you will lose body fat; you must eat fewer calories consistently to achieve this. If you eat only chicken, rice and broccoli but consume a higher quantity than you need, you'll still gain body fat despite eating clean, healthy, nutrient dense meals.

Banking calories.

Think about banking your calories like putting money away in a savings account. Say you're looking to save £70 each week. It does not matter whether you save £10 each day which will equate to your goal by the end of the week, or sporadically save different amounts each day. If by the end of the week you have saved £70, the result is the same. When it comes to calories; don't think of hitting your calories daily, think about it as a weekly goal. If your goal to lose 2lbs each week is to eat 1,800 calories, then your weekly target is 12,600. If you know you have a birthday night out on Saturday which you're going out for dinner and a few drinks do not stress! Reduce your calories slightly Monday to Friday and Sunday by 200 calories. This means you have an extra 1,200 calories to consume guilt free because at the end of the week you would have consumed the same amount to reduce your weight. By throwing in exercise a few times during the week will even further increase your energy expenditure for the week which means your rate of progress will be even quicker.

The main reason people overeat isn't because they are hungry all the time. It is important to identify the main reason you are overeating to break the mould, to break the habit and change your way of thinking in order to change. Here are a few examples someone might overeat.

• Same routine every night. Watching TV with a snack before bed.
• Struggling to say no when offered food.
• Not being prepared so opt for getting a takeaway for lunch and dinner.
• Having an ingrained belief that you must finish your plate because of starving kids in Africa.

- Snacks being in the cupboard.
- Boredom.
- Fatigue.
- Stress.
- Loneliness.
- An escape from reality.
- Quick source of joy.

If you are looking to break the mould, it's important to identify the reason you overeat which are known as trigger points. For example, if you know you snack at night because it has been part of your routine for so long you can break the mould by - Interrupting your routine by brushing your teeth after dinner, going to bed earlier, not buying as many snacks in the shop, or read a book instead of watching TV. When your routine doesn't change it'll be much more difficult to change. Most likely you associate the TV with a snack, or the computer with a cup of tea with a few biscuits. The TV or computer are your trigger points for food, even when you aren't hungry at all. When you eat it is important to be mindful of what goes in your body and to isolate yourself from your trigger point. Eating whilst doing another task will very easily lead to overeating without even realising. If you have an ingrained belief that you need to finish your plate because it offended your Granny when you were growing up, you must realise that it isn't the food you are wasting; it's yourself. By overeating you're wasting away your health, gaining excess weight which is the biggest waste of all.

For those who overeat because of emotional reasons such as sadness or low moods, it is important to remember excess food will only bring more sadness into your life by distilling guilt and anger. The initial pleasure you will experience will quickly vanish and to combat these emotions a vitious cycle can develop like dealing with the guilt of overeating by overeating more. Physically, your energy will dip very quickly if your blood sugar level spikes then dips making you feel tired, creating even lower mood and anger. The small sense of joy overeating will bring will be massively outweighed by the negative feelings you will experience straight after eating it.

Although you think you will only be happy when you lose four stone, at what cost will you go through to get there? If you hate the process, you'll be miserable. If you go on a crash diet, you'll not only be miserable, but you'll also be starving and be a grumpy prick with dangerously low energy levels. Once you get to your target weight will you be able to sustain it? Trying to sustain your new weight will most likely make you miserable. Years and years of binge eating means you have developed a habit of overeating. Breaking a habit doesn't go automatically just because you've had a health kick. That's why being smart, gradually losing a few pounds each week with a controlled calorie deficit with exercise you enjoy, increasing energy output will always be the best method for success. Replacing your night-time snacks with low calorie snacks are far more beneficial than going cold turkey because it is more sustainable. If you've lived the past ten years having a night-time snack; trying to cut it out entirely will drive you insane, no matter how much motivation you think you have.

Correlation vs Causation.

Social media is such a big platform, it seems like everyone has an opinion. This can be great because it has never been easier to get information about any topic as quickly. There are some really credible sources in a vast range of topics that share valuable and evidence-based information to help the reader in whatever subject they're looking for. However, it can also be an absolute mine field. Just because someone is dressed like a doctor in a video does not mean the information is correct. Or the number of followers somebody has does not correlate to how accurate their information they are preaching is. The more followers somebody has the chances are they are sponsored by certain products and are paid to promote them, despite what they may truly think about it. If you hear a "Study" being done and it seems too good to be true, especially to further push their message across, then it most likely is. Social media loves promoting quick fixes or drastic action with minimal effort, for a "Small fee."

Cigarettes are the causation of major life threatening diseases like cancer, heart disease, lung diseases, strokes, etc. Smoking directly causes a person to develop these diseases and can be avoided by stopping this habit. There is a lot of false information out there especially when it comes to our nutrition that correlates certain foods with health risks. Like studies showing that red meat will lead to a higher chance of a heart attack because their study showed the majority of people who suffered from heart attacks ate more red meat. In studies like these the author is usually trying to push their own agenda onto their readers, making it seem like red meat is the devil. It so happens that unhealthier people would consume more red meat in forms of highly processed and fatty burgers, steaks and pork chops. They usually neglect their overall health resulting in their inevitable heart attack. Red meat isn't the causation of their heart attack, it is a correlation.

To distinguish whether a product or study is correct you can either do your own research or ask yourself whether the results are due to correlation or did it have a direct causation. Like a study that shows watching TV causes obesity because most obese people spend more time watching tv; you must understand the television was not the cause of their obesity. Obese people will naturally spend more time being sedentary, therefore will watch more TV as a result. Another example is a bodybuilder promoting a brand-new protein product and insists his results are directly linked with this new product. Ignore the fact he is obviously paid to promote this product, his whole life is dedicated to being the best shape he possibly can and was probably doing bicep curls in the womb. Not everything is as it seems on social media, so please be careful what information you take in when scrolling through your news feed.

When trying to distinguish the truth in an article or study you must accept there are lucky anomaly's that will push their argument further because of the correlation of a product or act, as opposed to the causation. An anomaly is a very small minority that deviates from what is normal. Like reading an article about Sharon who miraculously recovered from her cataracts because she bought healing crystals or chanting Hare Krishna twenty times in-front of the mirror. This might be me being sceptical, but I don't correlate the improvement of her eyesight with her spiritual actions, but instead think the explanation can be due to something more scientific and logical. You can decide for yourself whether her affirmations and healing crystals were the causation of her healed eyes, or if she was an anomaly that linked the two together.

Or when Tony argues that his uncle is the fittest, healthiest person he knows despite the fact he smokes fifty cigarettes a day so therefore smoking does not cause any health risks. Tony's uncle in this case might have underlying health issues that he has not discovered yet, or is just an anomaly that has maintained his cardiovascular health despite his smoking habits.

Use it or lose it.

Once you get over the age of 65 you can lose up to 40% of your muscle mass. After the third decade of your life your body involuntarily and gradually loses muscle mass also known as sarcopenia. Unfortunately, there is no magical youth fountain that you can go to at the age of 65 and turn back time to re-live your youth. The only and best method to stay healthy by reducing sarcopenia is with resistance training. To continuously put your body under controlled stress for muscles to keep repairing and building. This means you won't struggle to get up off your seat, be able to get in and out of the bath with no issues, to still be fit enough to run after your kids and grandkids at a later stage of life. It is never too late to start a fitness journey. If anybody argues with you that they are too old to start a fitness journey let them know they are wrong!

Use it or lose it doesn't only represent physical ability, but it goes for your mental health, confidence, determination, tenacity and courage. If you don't constantly push yourself out of your comfort zone, you'll slowly lose your confidence in your abilities. If you've developed an injury and keep putting off playing football again, the confidence in your ability to play will shrink. Similarly, if you don't practice speaking in front of people, you'll lose your confidence to do so when giving a presentation in work. Psychological abilities must be consistently practiced just like physical fitness in order to develop and grow.

"Insanity is doing the same thing over and over again and expecting a different result." (Albert Einstein)

In order to develop your physical and mental health you must constantly push your boundaries. If you do the same thing repeatedly you will always remain the same. A fitness regime should always be constantly reviewed, be it your training programmes, weight, measurements, calorie consumption, body fat percentage etc. Unless these are constantly reviewed, you'll never know whether the work you are putting in is worth your while. If you are consistently checking your results and nothing is changing but you continue to do the same thing week after week, then you must change something otherwise you are literally wasting your time and energy.

Energy.

We only have a finite amount of time and energy in our lifetime. Be careful how you use these sources because they are the most precious things in life and the only things you can truly own. Think of your time as a bank account, but instead of getting paid each month and the balance being topped up, this account is only a finite number that can never be added to. Just like you'll not drain your bank account with buying things you don't need and you know you won't get any benefit from, do the same with your time and energy. Only invest in things that will benefit you. Even if you've been invested in something for a long time but you know it's draining your account, it's never too late to free yourself. Whether it be leaving a job you hate, a relationship you're not happy in, walking away from a toxic friend or family member that constantly puts you down, or stepping away from an environment that is damaging your health. Back yourself to succeed and be the happiest version you can be, even if nobody else does.

I beg you to start your side business that you've been dreaming of but have been putting off, or ask the guy or girl out for a date, or emigrate to that country you've been thinking about. What's the worst that can happen? If it does fail at least you tried. Sure, you might experience a bit of embarrassment and it might hurt your ego, but at least you'll not regret not giving it a go. Imagine if it does work out though. Imagine how much more fulfilled your life would be and how much happier you would become. Being in no relationship at all is far better than being in an unhappy one. Anyone who has been in a toxic relationship will truly understand you do not need a partner to be happy. Just because your friends are in relationships does not mean they are happier than you. Your friends or celebrities may post plenty of photos of themselves smiling and showing off how happy and perfect their lives are, but the reality is they might be feeling trapped or miserable. Posting selfies and videos of themselves on a night out to get acknowledgment from their peers isn't happiness. To me this shows desperation for validation. Getting nice comments is the only way to fuel their confidence due to their low self-esteem which may shock many people, but in my experience, this is the truth. Don't mistake noise as confidence. Generally, the loudest, chattiest people in the room are the least confident due to overcompensating for their true feelings. From my experience of coaching clients, it is clear that everybody has their own individual battles despite having a persona of true self-assurance.

When you take care of yourself, the more energy

you have to pass onto your friends and family. Taking care of yourself means physically looking after your health by exercising, fuelling your body with nutrient dense food and sleeping sufficiently. It also means looking after your emotional well-being by taking time for yourself to do what you enjoy and continuing to do the hobbies you love to do. Not doing things just to please other people, but really do something because you love it. I think too many relationships struggle because one person expects the other to mould into their way of life without considering the other partner. This person will lose their sense of purpose and forget their identity before they became a couple resulting in this person doing everything to please their partner despite what they may truly want. In my view; relationships, friendships and families should be about compromising with each other to keep everyone happy. Taking consideration and time to do what each other wants instead of expecting your partner to immediately fit into your ideology is the key to a long lasting, happy relationship.

You must balance your energy otherwise you will burn out. If you waste your energy on toxic, juvenile unimportant drama, you won't have the energy required to invest in yourself. Too many people waste their precious energy on people who don't deserve their time, leaving them exhausted with no return. If this resonates with you then you must do what you can to protect your energy so that can be used for better investments like your health, business and family. Stay well away from energy draining people because nothing good will come out of it, other than leaving you feeling utterly fed up and worn out.

PART 4

Closing statement

If you are serious about making a change to your life, take action now. Hopefully this book has inspired you to make some sort of change in at least one aspect of your life. Inspiration means nothing without taking action which is the only means of growth in your life. Remember, being inspired leads to motivation which can quickly run out and therefore nothing will be done. Don't wait until next week, or even next year. There is never a perfect time to start other than right now. Contact a friend or coach to kick start your fitness journey, start journalling today, or go to the grocery store to start meal prepping instead of getting a takeaway tonight. Interrupt your usual habits by changing your weekly routine with new, exciting and challenging habits to direct you to where you want to be.

This book can either be a mixture of words bunched together to make random, non-provoking, meaningless sentences. Or it can really be the fire you needed to finally make that change in your life you've always wanted to make but have been putting off until the "Perfect time." Motivational quotes can just be a few irrelevant words jumbled together that you'll scroll past on your news feed without a second thought, or you can take a second to reflect on these words, relate the quote to your own circumstances and put them into action. You can read something like "Believe in yourself," and think how silly and generic that is because you've heard it a million times before. But when you reflect on your own life, it can quite literally change your life, depending on your mind set and whether you really want to make a change or not will depend on how much of an effect this book will have on you.

Being productive VS being busy are very different things. Productivity drives you forward and gets you that step further to reaching your goals. Being busy on the other hand keeps you occupied without making any progress. You can be busy procrastinating, doing things that don't need to be done like scrolling through your phone or sorting out your cupboards in your kitchen to distract yourself from what needs to be done. My mission for you is to plan out each day in order to be productive and to make progress regarding your ambitions, hopes and dreams. It can be too easy to make yourself busy without doing anything meaningful, so set yourself small tasks each day and consistently build on it to get to where you'd love to be.

This December 31st when you reflect on the year behind you, will you regret the decisions you didn't do? Have you accomplished the goals you set yourself this time last year? Or has it been just another year of remaining in the exact same spot as last year? What will it take for you to finally do what you've always wanted to do? If upon reflection you are happy with your achievements over the last 12 months then I'm proud of you, as you should be too. If you're not however, let this be the last year this will ever happen. No more willy nilly New Year's resolutions, no more dreaming about something that one day will miraculously happen to you. This is the time to change.

From the bottom of my heart, thank you so much for getting to the end of my book. I purposefully made it quite short because I didn't want to fill the book with anything that didn't need to be in it. If you even feel a little bit inspired to do something that'll benefit you in any way, just go for it. You'll always regret the things you don't do or say rather than the things you do. Think positively about the future rather than always fearing the worst because this is what usually leads to not even giving it a go. Back yourself to win. If nobody else believes in you, I do.

CPSIA information can be obtained
at www.ICGtesting.com
Printed in the USA
BVHW032251161122
652180BV00011B/122

9 798358 894129